The Essential Air Fryer Toaster Oven Recipe Book

A Complete Collection Of Side Dishes to Boost Your Air Fryer Toaster Oven Meals

Eva Morris

TABLE OF CONTENT

medical or professional advice. The content within this book has been derived from various sources. Please consult a licensed professional before attempting any techniques outlined in this book.

By reading this document, the reader agrees that under no circumstances is the author responsible for any losses, direct or indirect, which are incurred as a result of the use of information contained within this document, including, but not limited to, — errors, omissions, or inaccuracies.

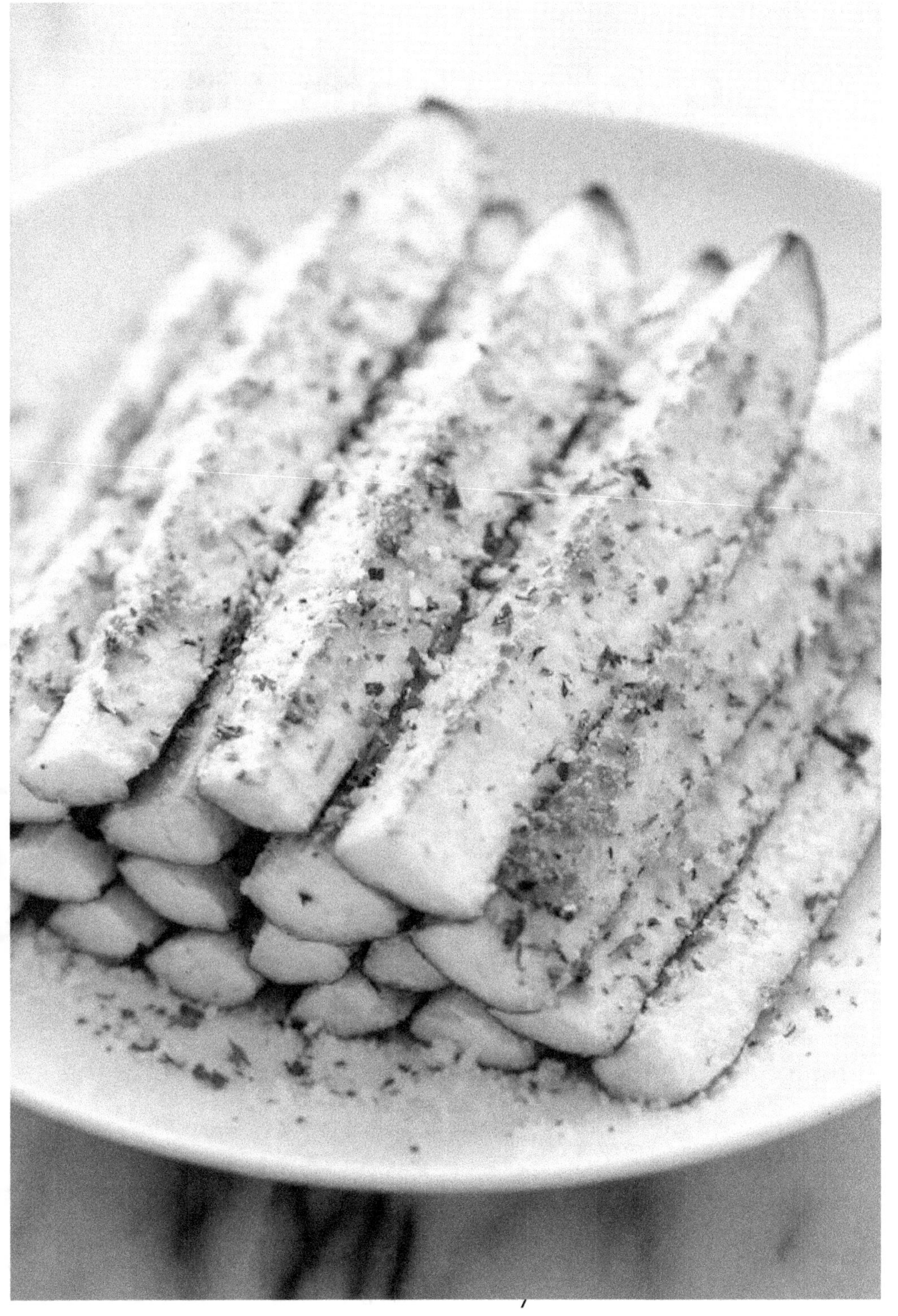

Chicken Thighs With Butternut Squash

Preparation Time: 10 minutes

Cooking time: 30 minutes

Servings: 6

Ingredients:

- 3cups butternut squash, cubed
- Six boneless chicken thighs
- A sprig of fresh sage, chopped
- 1tbsp olive oil
- Salt and pepper to taste

Directions:

1. Preheat the oven to 4250F.

2. In a skillet, sauté the butternut squash and season with salt and pepper to taste. Once the squash is cooked, remove from the skillet and set aside.

3. Using the same skillet, add oil and cook the chicken thighs for 10 minutes on each side.

4. Season with salt and pepper, and add the squash back.

5. Remove the skillet from the stove and bake in the oven for 15 minutes.

6. Serve and enjoy.

Nutrition:

Calories 300, Total Fat 13g, Saturated Fat 3.5g, Total Carbs 9g, Net Carbs 7.5g, Protein 35g, Sugar: 2g, Fiber 1.5g, Sodium 149mg, Potassium 640mg

Cajun Rice & Chicken

Preparation Time: 10 minutes

Cooking time: 20 minutes

Servings: 6

Ingredients:

- One tablespoon oil
- One onion, diced
- Three cloves of garlic, minced
- 1-pound chicken breasts, sliced
- One tablespoon Cajun seasoning
- One tablespoon tomato paste
- cups chicken broth
- 1½ cups brown rice, rinsed
- One bell pepper, chopped

Directions:

1. Place a heavy-bottomed pot on medium-high fire and heat for 2 minutes.

2. Add oil and heat for a minute.

3. Sauté the onion and garlic until fragrant.

4. Stir in the chicken breasts and season with Cajun seasoning.

5. Continue cooking for 3 minutes.

6. Add the tomato paste, rice, and chicken broth. Bring to a boil while stirring to dissolve the tomato paste.

7. Once boiling, lower fire to a simmer, cover, and cook until liquid is fully absorbed, around 15 minutes.

8. Turn off the fire and let it stand for another 5 minutes before serving.

Nutrition:

Calories 224, Total Fat 6g, Saturated Fat 1.3g, Total Carbs 16g, Net Carbs 14g, Protein 26g, Sugar: 2g, Fiber 2g, Sodium 646mg, Potassium 339mg

Parmesan Zucchini Rounds

Preparation Time: 25 minutes

Cooking Time: 20 minutes

Servings: 4

Ingredients:

- Four zucchinis; sliced

- 1 ½ cups parmesan; grated

- ¼ cup parsley; chopped.

- One egg whisked

- One egg white; whisked

- ½ tsp. garlic powder

- Cooking spray

Directions:

1. Take a bowl and mix the egg with egg whites, parmesan, parsley, and garlic powder and whisk.

2. Dredge each zucchini slice in this mix, place them all in your air fryer's basket, grease them with cooking spray and cook at 370°F for 20 minutes

3. Divide between plates and serve as a side dish.

Nutrition:

Calories: 183

Fat 6g

Fiber 2g

Carbs: 3g

Protein 8g

Green Bean Casserole

Preparation Time: 25 minutes

Cooking Time: 20 minutes

Servings: 4

Ingredients:

- 1 lb. fresh green beans, edges trimmed

- ½ oz. pork rinds, finely ground

- 1 oz. full-Fat cream cheese

- ½ cup heavy whipping cream

- ¼ cup diced yellow onion

- ½ cup chopped white mushrooms

- ½ cup chicken broth

- 4 tbsp. unsalted butter.

- ¼ tsp. xanthan gum

Directions:

1. In a medium saucepan over medium heat, melt the butter. Sauté onion and mushrooms until smooth and fragrant. Do it for about 3-5 minutes.

2. Add thick cream, cream cheese, and stock to skillet. Whisk until smooth. Bring to a boil and then simmer. Pour the blonde chewing gum into the pan and remove from the heat

3. Cut the green beans into 2-inch pieces and place them in a 4-cup round skillet. Pour sauce mixture over them and stir until covered. Fill the plate with ground pork rind. Place in the fryer basket

4. Set the temperature to 320 degrees F and set the timer for 15 minutes. The top will be green and gold beans when fully cooked. Serve hot.

Nutrition:

Calories: 267

Protein 3.6g

Fat 23.4g

Carbs: 9.7g

Zucchini Spaghetti

Preparation Time: 20 minutes

Cooking Time: 15 minutes

Servings: 4

Ingredients:

- 1 lb. zucchinis cut with a paralyzer
- One cup parmesan; grated
- ¼ cup parsley; chopped.
- ¼ cup olive oil
- Six garlic cloves; minced
- ½ tsp. red pepper flakes
- Salt
- Black pepper

Directions:

In a pan that fits your air fryer, mix all the ingredients, toss, introduce in the fryer, and cook at 370°F for 15 minutes. Divide between plates and serve as a side dish.

Nutrition:

Calories: 200

Fat 6g

Carbs: 4g

Protein 5g

Cabbage And Radishes Mix

Preparation Time: 20 minutes

Cooking Time: 15 minutes

Servings: 4

Ingredients:

- Six cups green cabbage; shredded
- ½ cup celery leaves; chopped.
- ¼ cup green onions; chopped.
- Six radishes; sliced
- 3 tbsp. olive oil
- 2 tbsp. Balsamic vinegar
- ½ tsp. Hot paprika
- 1tsp. lemon juice

Directions:

1. In your skillet, combine all ingredients and pour well.

2. Place skillet in a deep fryer and cook at 380 ° F for 15 minutes. Divide between dishes and serve as a dish.

Nutrition:

Calories: 130

Fat 4g

Carbs: 4g

Protein 7g

Jicama Fries

Preparation Time: 30 minutes

Cooking Time: 20 minutes

Servings: 4

Ingredients:

- One small jicama, peeled.
- ¼ tsp. Onion powder
- ¾tsp. Chili powder
- ¼ tsp. ground black pepper
- ¼ tsp. garlic powder

Directions:

1. Cut jicama into matchstick-sized pieces.
2. Place pieces into a small bowl and sprinkle with remaining ingredients. Place the fries into the air fryer basket
3. Adjust the temperature to 350 Degrees F and set the timer for 20 minutes. Toss the basket two or three times during cooking. Serve warm.

Nutrition:

Calories: 37

Protein 0.8g

Fat 0.1g

Carbs: 8.7g

Kale Chips

Preparation Time: 10 minutes

Cooking Time: 5 minutes

Servings: 4

Ingredients:

- Four cups stemmed kale
- ½ tsp. salt
- 2 tsp. avocado oil

Directions:

1. Take a large bowl, toss the kale in avocado oil and sprinkle with salt. Place into the air fryer basket.

2. Adjust the temperature to 400 Degrees F and set the timer for 5 minutes. Kale will be crispy when done. Serve immediately.

Nutrition:

Calories: 25

Protein 0.5g

Fat 2.2g

Carbs: 1.1g

Coriander Artichokes

Preparation Time: 20 minutes

Cooking Time: 15 minutes

Servings: 4

Ingredients:

- 12 oz. artichoke hearts
- 1 tbsp. lemon juice
- 1 tsp. Coriander, ground
- ½ tsp. Cumin seeds
- ½ tsp. olive oil
- Salt and black pepper

Directions:

1. In a pan that fits your air fryer, mix all the ingredients, toss, introduce the pan in the fryer, and cook at 370°F for 15 minutes. Divide the mix between plates and serve as a side dish.

Nutrition:

Calories: 200

Fat 7g

Carbs: 5g

Protein 8g

Spinach And Artichokes Sauté

Preparation Time: 20 minutes

Cooking Time: 15 minutes

Servings: 4

Ingredients:

- 10 oz. artichoke hearts; halved
- 2 cups baby spinach
- Three garlic cloves
- ¼ cup veggie stock
- 2 tsp. lime juice
- Salt and black pepper

Directions:

1. In a pan that fits your air fryer, mix all the ingredients, toss, introduce in the fryer, and cook at 370°F for 15 minutes. Divide between plates and serve as a side dish.

Nutrition:

Calories: 209

Fat 6g

Carbs: 4g

Protein 8g

Green Beans

Preparation Time: 5 minutes

Cooking Time: 20 minutes

Servings: 4

Ingredients:

- 6 cups green beans; trimmed
- 1 tbsp. hot paprika
- 2 tbsp. olive oil
- A pinch of salt and black pepper

Directions:

1. Take a bowl, mix the beans with the other ingredients, toss them, put them in the fryer basket, and cook at 370 ° F for 20 minutes.

2. Divide between dishes and serve as a garnish.

Nutrition:

Calories: 120

Fat 5g

Carbs: 4g

Protein 2g

Balsamic Cabbage

Preparation Time: 10 minutes

Cooking Time: 15 minutes

Servings: 4

Ingredients:

- 6 cups red cabbage; shredded
- Four garlic cloves; minced
- 1 tbsp. olive oil
- 1 tbsp. balsamic vinegar
- Salt and black pepper

Directions:

1. In a frying pan that fits the deep fryer, combine all ingredients, mix, place skillet in the deep fryer, and cook at 380 ° F for 15 minutes. Divide between dishes and serve as a garnish.

Nutrition:

Calories: 151

Fat 2g

Carbs: 5g

Protein 5g

Herbed Radish Sauté

Preparation Time: 5 minutes

Cooking Time: 15 minutes

Servings: 4

Ingredients:

- Two bunches red radishes; halved
- 2 tbsp. Parsley, chopped.
- 2 tbsp. balsamic vinegar
- 1 tbsp. olive oil
- Salt and black pepper

Directions:

1. Take a bowl and mix the radishes with the remaining ingredients except for the parsley, toss and put them in your air fryer's basket.

2. Cook at 400°F for 15 minutes, divide between plates, sprinkle the parsley on top and serve as a side dish

Nutrition:

Calories: 180

Fat 4g

Carbs: 3g

Protein 5g

Roasted Tomatoes

Preparation Time: 5 minutes

Cooking Time: 15 minutes

Servings: 4

Ingredients:

- Four tomatoes; halved

- ½ cup parmesan; grated

- 1 tbsp. basil; chopped.

- ½ tsp. Onion powder

- ½ tsp. Oregano; dried

- ½ tsp. Smoked paprika

- ½ tsp. garlic powder

- Cooking spray

Directions:

1. Get a bowl and add up all the ingredients except the cooking spray and the parmesan.

2. Arrange the tomatoes in your air fryer's pan, sprinkle the parmesan on top, and

grease with cooking spray

3. Cook at 370°F for 15 minutes, divide between plates, and serve.

Nutrition:

Calories: 200

Fat 7g

Carbs: 4g

Protein 6g

Kale And Walnuts

Preparation Time: 5 minutes

Cooking Time: 15 minutes

Servings: 4

Ingredients:

- Three garlic cloves
- 10 cups kale; roughly chopped
- 1/3 cup parmesan; grated
- ½ cup almond milk
- ¼ cup walnuts; chopped.
- 1 tbsp. Butter; melted
- ¼ tsp. nutmeg, ground
- Salt and black pepper

Directions:

1. In a pan that fits the air fryer, combine all the ingredients, toss, introduce the pan in the machine and cook at 360°F for 15 minutes
2. Divide between plates and serve.

Nutrition:

Calories: 160

Fat 7g

Carbs: 4g

Protein 5g

Bok Choy And Butter Sauce

Preparation Time: 5 minutes

Cooking Time: 15 minutes

Servings: 4

Ingredients:

- Two bok Choy heads; trimmed and cut into strips
- 1 tbsp. butter; melted
- 2 tbsp. chicken stock
- 1 tsp. lemon juice
- 1 tbsp. olive oil
- A pinch of salt and black pepper

Directions:

1. In a pan that fits your air fryer, mix all the ingredients, toss, introduce the pan in the air fryer, and cook at 380°F for 15 minutes. Divide between plates and serve as a side dish

Nutrition:

Calories: 141

Fat 3g

Carbs: 4g

Protein 3g

Turmeric Mushroom

Preparation Time: 5 minutes

Cooking Time: 15 minutes

Servings: 4

Ingredients:

- 1 lb. brown mushrooms
- Four garlic cloves; minced
- ¼ tsp. cinnamon powder
- 1 tsp. Olive oil
- ½ tsp. turmeric powder
- Salt and black pepper to taste

Directions:

1. In a bowl, combine all the ingredients and toss.
2. Put the mushrooms in your air fryer's basket and cook at 370°F for 15 minutes
3. Divide the mix between plates and serve as a side dish.

Nutrition:

Calories: 208

Fat 7g

Carbs: 5g

Protein 7g

Baked Vegetables

Preparation Time: 10 minutes

Cooking Time: 30 minutes

Serve: 6

Ingredients:

- Two zucchini, sliced
- Two tomatoes, quartered
- Six fresh basil leaves, sliced
- 2 tsp. Italian seasoning
- 2 tbsp. olive oil
- One eggplant, sliced
- One onion, sliced
- One bell pepper, cut into strips
- Pepper
- Salt

Directions:

1. Fit the Cuisinart oven with the rack in position 1.

2. Add all ingredients except basil leaves into the bowl and toss well.

3. Transfer vegetable mixture to parchment-lined baking pan.

4. Set to bake at 400 F for 35 minutes. After 5 minutes, place the baking pan in the preheated oven.

5. Garnish with basil and serve.

Nutrition:

Calories 96

Fat 5.5 g

Carbohydrates 11.7 g

Sugar 6.4 g

Protein 2.3 g

Cholesterol 1 mg

Cheese Herb Zucchini

Preparation Time: 10 minutes

Cooking Time: 15 minutes

Serve: 4

Ingredients:

- Four zucchini, quartered
- 1/2 tsp. dried oregano
- 2 tbsp. fresh parsley, chopped
- 2 tbsp. olive oil
- 1/2 tsp. dried thyme
- 1/2 cup parmesan cheese, grated
- 1/4 tsp. garlic powder
- 1/2 tsp. dried basil
- Pepper
- Salt

Directions:

1. Fit the Cuisinart oven with the rack in position 1.

2. In a small bowl, mix parmesan cheese, garlic powder, basil, oregano, thyme, pepper, and salt.

3. Arrange zucchini in baking pan and drizzle with oil, and sprinkle with parmesan cheese mixture.

4. Set to bake at 350 F for 20 minutes. After 5 minutes, place the baking pan in the preheated oven.

5. Garnish with parsley and serve.

Nutrition:

Calories 130

Fat 9.8 g

Carbohydrates 7.4 g

Sugar 3.5 g

Protein 6.1 g

Cholesterol 8 mg

Healthy Spinach Muffins

Preparation Time: 10 minutes

Cooking Time: 15 minutes

Serve: 12

Ingredients:

- Ten eggs

- 2 cups spinach, chopped

- 1/2 tsp. dried basil

- 1 1/2 cups parmesan cheese, grated

- 1/4 tsp. garlic powder

- 1/4 tsp. onion powder

- Salt

Directions:

1. Fit the Cuisinart oven with the rack in position 1.

2. Spray 12-cups muffin tin with cooking spray and set aside.

3. In a large bowl, whisk eggs with basil, garlic powder, onion powder, and salt.

4. Add cheese and spinach and stir well.

5. Pour egg mixture into the prepared muffin tin.

6. Set to bake at 400 F for 20 minutes. After 5 minutes, place the muffin tin in the preheated oven.

7. Serve and enjoy.

Nutrition:

Calories 90

Fat 6.1 g

Carbohydrates 0.9 g

Sugar 0.3 g

Protein 8.4 g

Cholesterol 144 mg

Honey Corn Muffins

Preparation Time: 10 minutes

Cooking Time: 20 minutes

Serve: 8

Ingredients:

- Two eggs

- 1/2 cup sugar

- 1 1/4 cups self-rising flour

- 3/4 cup yellow cornmeal

- 1/2 cup butter, melted

- 3/4 cup buttermilk

- 1 tbsp. honey

Directions:

1. Fit the Cuisinart oven with the rack in position 1.

2. Spray 8-cups muffin tin with cooking spray and set aside.

3. In a large bowl, mix cornmeal, sugar, and flour.

4. In a separate bowl, whisk the eggs with buttermilk and honey until well combined.

5. Slowly add egg mixture and melted butter to the cornmeal mixture and stir until just mixed.

6. Spoon batter into the prepared muffin tin.

7. Set to bake at 350 F for 25 minutes. After 5 minutes, place the muffin tin in the preheated oven.

8. Serve and enjoy.

Nutrition:

Calories 294

Fat 13.4 g

Carbohydrates 39.6 g

Sugar 16 g

Protein 5.2 g

Cholesterol 72 mg

Delicious Mac And Cheese

Preparation Time: 10 minutes

Cooking Time: 30 minutes

Serve: 6

Ingredients:

- 2 1/2 cups pasta, uncooked

- 1/2 cup cream

- 1 cup vegetable broth

- 2 tbsp. flour

- 1/2 cup parmesan cheese, grated

- 1/2 cup Velveeta cheese, cut into small cubes

- 2 cups Colby cheese, shredded

- 2 tbsp. butter

- 1 tsp. salt

Directions:

1. Fit the Cuisinart oven with the rack in position 1.

2. Cook pasta according to the packet instructions. Drain well.

3. Melt butter in a pan over medium heat. Slowly whisk in flour.

4. Whisk constantly and slowly add the broth.

5. Slowly pour the cream and whisk constantly.

6. Slowly add parmesan cheese, Velveeta cheese, and Colby cheese and whisk until smooth.

7. Add cooked pasta to the sauce and stir well to coat.

8. Transfer pasta into the greased casserole dish.

9. Set to bake at 350 F for 35 minutes. After 5 minutes, place the casserole dish in the preheated oven.

10. Serve and enjoy.

Nutrition:

Calories 410

Fat 21.8 g

Carbohydrates 34 g

Sugar 1.3 g

Protein 20 g

Cholesterol 99 mg

Jalapeno Bread

Preparation Time: 10 minutes

Cooking Time: 50 minutes

Serve: 10

Ingredients:

- 3 cups all-purpose flour
- 8 oz. cheddar cheese, shredded
- 1/2 tsp. ground white pepper
- 1 1/2 tbsp. baking powder
- 1/4 cup butter, melted
- 1 1/2 cups buttermilk
- Three jalapeno peppers, chopped
- 2 tbsp. sugar
- 1 1/4 tsp. salt

Directions:

1. Fit the Cuisinart oven with the rack in position 1.

2. In a mixing bowl, mix flour, baking powder, sugar, white pepper, and salt.

3. Add jalapenos and cheese and stir to combine.

4. Whisk butter and buttermilk together and add to the flour mixture. Stir until just combined.

5. Pour batter into the greased 9*5-inch loaf pan.

6. Set to bake at 375 F for 55 minutes. After 5 minutes, place the loaf pan in the preheated oven.

7. Slice and serve.

Nutrition:

Calories 297

Fat 12.9 g

Carbohydrates 34.5 g

Sugar 4.5 g

Protein 10.9 g

Cholesterol 37 mg

Healthy Barley Bread

Preparation Time: 10 minutes

Cooking Time: 40 minutes

Serve: 16

Ingredients:

- Two eggs
- 1/2 tsp. baking soda
- 2 tbsp. baking powder
- 3 cups barley flour
- 3 tbsp. honey
- 1/3 cup olive oil
- 1 1/2 cups buttermilk
- 1 1/4 tsp. salt

Directions:

1. Fit the Cuisinart oven with the rack in position 1.

2. In a large bowl, mix flour, baking powder, baking soda, and salt.

3. In a separate bowl, whisk eggs with honey, oil, and buttermilk.

4. Add egg mixture into the flour mixture and stir until just combined.

5. Pour batter into the greased loaf pan.

6. Set to bake at 350 F for 40 minutes. After 5 minutes, place the loaf pan in the preheated oven.

7. Slice and serve.

Nutrition:

Calories 163

Fat 5.4 g

Carbohydrates 26 g

Sugar 4.6 g

Protein 4.4 g

Cholesterol 21 mg

Rice Broccoli Casserole

Preparation Time: 10 minutes

Cooking Time: 40 minutes

Serve: 8

Ingredients:

- 2 cups brown rice, cooked
- 3 cups broccoli florets
- 1 tbsp. olive oil
- Two garlic cloves, minced
- One onion, chopped

For sauce:

- 1tbsp onion, chopped
- 1/4 cup nutritional yeast flakes
- 1cup of water
- 1garlic clove, minced
- 1tbsp tapioca starch
- 1cup cashews
- 1 1/2 tsp. salt

Directions:

1. Fit the Cuisinart oven with the rack in position 1.

2. For the sauce: add all sauce ingredients into the blender and blend until smooth.

3. Heat oil in a pan over medium-high heat.

4. Add garlic and onion and sauté until onion is softened.

5. Add broccoli and cook for a minute.

6. Add rice and sauce and stir to combine.

7. Transfer broccoli rice mixture into the greased casserole dish.

8. Set to bake at 400 F for 45 minutes. After 5 minutes, place the casserole dish in the preheated oven.

9. Serve and enjoy.

Nutrition:

Calories 327

Fat 11.4 g

Carbohydrates 49.2 g

Sugar 2.1 g

Protein 9.7 g

Cholesterol 0 mg

Tomato And Beef Sauce

Preparation Time: 25 minutes

Cooking Time: 20 minutes

Serving: 4

Ingredients:

- 1lb. Lean beef meat; cubed and browned
- 16oz. Tomato sauce
- 2garlic cloves; minced
- Cooking spray
- Salt and black pepper to taste.

Directions:

1. Preheat the air fryer at 400°f, add the pan inside, grease it with cooking spray, add the meat and all the other ingredients, toss and cook for 20 minutes
2. Divide into bowls and serve.

Nutrition: calories: 270; fat: 15g; fiber: 3g; carbs: 6g; protein: 12g

Eggplant Bake

Preparation Time: 25 minutes

Cooking Time: 20 minutes

Serving: 4

Ingredients:

- ½ lb. Cherry tomatoes; cubed
- ½ cup cilantro; chopped.
- Four garlic cloves; minced
- Two eggplants; cubed
- One hot chili pepper; chopped.
- Four spring onions; chopped.
- 2tsp. Olive oil
- Salt and black pepper to

Directions:

1. Grease a baking pan that fits the air fryer with the oil and mix all the pan ingredients.

2. Put the pan in the preheated air fryer and cook at 380°f for 20 minutes, divide into bowls and serve

Nutrition:

Calories: 232; fat: 12g; fiber: 3g; carbs: 5g; protein: 10g

Thyme Eggplant And Green Beans

Preparation Time: 25 minutes

Cooking Time: 20 minutes

Serving: 6

Ingredients:

- lb. Green beans; trimmed and halved
- Two eggplants; cubed
- One red bell pepper; chopped.
- 1 cup veggie stock
- One red chili pepper
- 1 tbsp. Olive oil
- ½ tsp. Thyme; dried
- Salt and black pepper

Directions:

1. In a pan that fits your air fryer, mix all the ingredients, toss, introduce the pan in the machine and cook at 350°f for 20 minutes

2. Divide into bowls and serve.

Nutrition:

Calories: 180; fat: 3g; fiber: 2g; carbs: 5g; protein: 7g

Garlicky Pork Stew

Preparation Time: 30 minutes

Cooking Time: 20 minutes

Serving: 4

Ingredients:

- 1 lb. Pork stew meat; cubed
- ¼ cup tomato sauce
- 1cup spinach; torn
- Three garlic cloves; minced
- ½ tsp. Olive oil

Directions:

1. In a pan that fits your air fryer, mix the pork with the other ingredients except for the spinach, toss, introduce in the fryer and cook at 370°f for 15 minutes

2. Add the spinach, toss, cook for 10 minutes more, divide into bowls and serve.

Nutrition: calories: 290; fat: 14g; fiber: 3g; carbs: 5g; protein: 13g

Tomatoes And Cabbage Stew

Preparation Time: 10 minutes

Cooking Time: 25 minutes

Serving: 4

Ingredients:

- 14 oz. Canned tomatoes; chopped.

- One green cabbage head; shredded

- 4 oz. chicken stock

- 2 tbsp. Dill; chopped.

- 1 tbsp. sweet paprika

- Salt and black pepper

Directions:

1. In a pan that fits your air fryer, mix the cabbage with the tomatoes and all the other ingredients except the dill, toss, introduce the pan in the fryer and cook at

380°F for 20 minutes

2. Divide into bowls and serve with dill sprinkled on top.

Nutrition: Calories: 200; Fat: 8g; Fiber: 3g; Carbs: 4g; Protein: 6g

Spinach And Shrimp

Preparation Time: 10 minutes

Cooking Time: 20 minutes

Serving: 4

Ingredients:

- 15 oz. shrimp; peeled and deveined
- ¼ cup veggie stock
- Two tomatoes; cubed
- Four spring onions; chopped.
- 2 cups baby spinach
- 1 tbsp. garlic; minced
- 2 tbsp. Cilantro; chopped.
- 1 tbsp. Lemon juice
- ½ tsp. cumin, ground
- Salt and black pepper to taste.

Directions:

1. In a pan that fits your air fryer, mix all the ingredients except the cilantro, toss, introduce in the air fryer and cook at 360°F for 15 minutes

2. Add the cilantro, stir, and divide into bowls.

Nutrition: Calories: 201; Fat: 8g; Fiber: 2g; Carbs: 4g; Protein: 8g

Fennel And Tomato Stew

Preparation Time: 10 minutes

Cooking Time: 25 minutes

Serving: 4

Ingredients:

- Two fennel bulbs; shredded

- ½ cup chicken stock

- One red bell pepper; chopped.

- Two garlic cloves; minced

- 2 cups tomatoes; cubed

- 2 tbsp. tomato puree

- 1 tsp. rosemary; dried

- 1 tsp. sweet paprika

- Salt and black pepper to taste.

Directions:

1. In a pan that fits your air fryer, mix all the ingredients, toss, introduce in the fryer and cook at 380°F for 15 minutes

2. Divide the stew into bowls.

Nutrition: Calories: 184; Fat: 7g; Fiber: 2g; Carbs: 3g; Protein: 8g

Courgettes Casserole

Preparation Time: 10 minutes

Cooking Time: 25 minutes

Serving: 4

Ingredients:

- 14 oz. cherry tomatoes; cubed
- Two spring onions; chopped.
- Three garlic cloves; minced
- Two courgettes; sliced
- Two celery sticks; sliced
- One yellow bell pepper; chopped.
- ½ cup mozzarella; shredded
- 1 tbsp. thyme; dried
- 1 tbsp. olive oil
- 1 tsp. smoked paprika

Directions:

1. In a baking dish that fits your air fryer, mix all the ingredients except the cheese and toss.

2. Sprinkle the cheese on top, introduce the dish in your air fryer and cook at 380°F for 20 minutes. Divide between plates and serve for lunch

Nutrition: Calories: 254; Fat: 12g; Fiber: 2g; Carbs: 4g; Protein: 11g

Basil Chicken Bites

Preparation Time: 10 minutes

Cooking Time: 30 minutes

Serving: 4

Ingredients:

- 1 ½ lb. chicken breasts, skinless; boneless and cubed

- ½ cup chicken stock

- ½ tsp. basil; dried

- 2 tsp. smoked paprika

- Salt and black pepper to taste.

Directions:

1. In a pan that fits the air fryer, combine all the ingredients, toss, introduce the pan in the fryer and cook at 390°F for 25 minutes

2. Divide between plates and serve for lunch with a side salad.

Nutrition: Calories: 223; Fat: 12g; Fiber: 2g; Carbs: 5g;
Protein: 13g

Paprika Cod

Preparation Time: 10 minutes

Cooking Time: 17 minutes

Serving: 4

Ingredients:

- 1 lb. cod fillets, boneless, skinless, and cubed

- One spring onion; chopped.

- 2 cups baby arugula

- 2 tbsp. Fresh cilantro; minced

- ½ tsp. Sweet paprika

- ½ tsp. oregano, ground

- A drizzle of olive oil

- Salt and black pepper to taste.

Directions:

1. Take a bowl and mix the cod with salt, pepper, paprika, oregano, and the oil, toss, transfer the cubes to your air fryer's basket

and cook at 360°F for 12 minutes

2. In a salad bowl, mix the cod with the remaining ingredients, toss, divide between plates and serve.

Nutrition: Calories: 240; Fat: 11g; Fiber: 3g; Carbs: 5g; Protein: 8g

Turkey And Mushroom Stew

Preparation Time: 10 minutes

Cooking Time: 30 minutes

Serving: 4

Ingredients:

- ½ lb. brown mushrooms; sliced
- One turkey breast, skinless, boneless; cubed and browned
- ¼ cup tomato sauce
- 1 tbsp. Parsley, chopped.
- Salt and black pepper

Directions:

1. In a pan that fits your air fryer, mix the turkey with the mushrooms, salt, pepper, and tomato sauce toss, introduce to the fryer and cook at 350°F for 25 minutes

2. Divide into bowls and serve for lunch with parsley sprinkled on top.

Nutrition: Calories: 220; Fat: 12g; Fiber: 2g; Carbs: 5g; Protein: 12g

Okra Casserole

Preparation Time: 10 minutes

Cooking Time: 20 minutes

Serving: 4

Ingredients:

- Two red bell peppers; cubed
- Two tomatoes; chopped.
- Three garlic cloves; minced
- 3 cups okra
- ½ cup cheddar; shredded
- ¼ cup tomato puree
- 1 tbsp. Cilantro; chopped.
- 1 tsp. olive oil
- 2 tsp. coriander, ground
- Salt and black pepper to taste.

Directions:

1. Grease a heatproof dish that fits your air fryer with the oil add all the ingredients except the cilantro and the cheese, and toss them gently

2. Sprinkle the cheese and the cilantro on top, introduce the dish in the fryer and cook at 390°F for 20 minutes.

3. Divide between plates and serve for lunch.

Nutrition: Calories: 221; Fat: 7g; Fiber: 2g; Carbs: 4g; Protein: 9g

Tomato And Avocado

Preparation Time: 5 minutes

Cooking Time: 8 minutes

Serving: 4

Ingredients:

- ½ lb. cherry tomatoes; halved
- Two avocados, pitted; peeled, and cubed
- One ¼ cup lettuce; torn
- 1/3 cup coconut cream
- A pinch of salt and black pepper
- Cooking spray

Directions:

1. Grease the air fryer with cooking spray, combine the tomatoes with avocados, salt, pepper, and the cream, and cook at 350°F for 5 minutes, shaking once

2. In a salad bowl, mix the lettuce with the tomatoes and avocado mix, toss and

serve.

Nutrition: Calories: 226; Fat: 12g; Fiber: 2g; Carbs: 4g; Protein: 8g

Turkey And Broccoli Stew

Preparation Time: 10 minutes

Cooking Time: 30 minutes

Serving: 4

Ingredients:

- One broccoli head, florets separated
- One turkey breast, skinless; boneless, and cubed
- 1 cup tomato sauce
- 1 tbsp. Parsley, chopped.
- 1 tbsp. olive oil
- Salt and black pepper

Directions:

1. In a baking dish that fits your air fryer, mix the turkey with the rest of the ingredients except the parsley, toss, introduce the plate in the fryer, bake at 380°F for 25 minutes

2. Divide into bowls, sprinkle the parsley on top, and serve.

Nutrition: Calories: 250; Fat: 11g; Fiber: 2g; Carbs: 6g; Protein: 12g

Rosemary Grilled Chicken

Preparation Time: 10 minutes

Cooking time: 10 minutes

Servings: 4

Ingredients:

- One teaspoon sea salt

- One tablespoon fresh parsley, finely chopped

- One tablespoon fresh rosemary, finely chopped

- One tablespoon olive oil

- Five cloves garlic, minced

- Four pieces of 6-oz chicken breast, boneless and skinless

Directions:

1. In a shallow and large bowl, mix salt, parsley, rosemary, olive oil, and garlic. Place chicken breast and marinate in a bowl of herbs for at least an hour or more

before grilling.

2. Grease grill grates and preheat grill to medium-high. Once hot, grill chicken for 4 to 5 minutes per side or until juices run a transparent and internal chicken temperature is 168oF.

Nutrition:

Calories 317, Total Fat 9g, Saturated Fat 2.2g, Total Carbs 1g, Net Carbs 0.8g, Protein 53g, Sugar: 0g, Fiber 0.2g, Sodium 709mg, Potassium 459mg

Curried Coconut Chicken

Preparation Time: 10 minutes

Cooking time: 40 minutes

Servings: 6

Ingredients:

- Four large tomatoes, sliced
- One can make coconut milk (14 -oz)
- Six cloves garlic, crushed then minced
- One whole onion, sliced thinly
- 1tbsp curry
- 1 tbsp. turmeric
- 1 tsp. cinnamon
- 1 tsp. clove powder
- 1 tsp. fenugreek
- 1-inch long ginger around thumb-sized, peeled
- Two bay leaves

- • 1/2 tsp. salt

- • 1 tsp. pepper

- • 2tbsp olive oil

- • 2lbs. boneless and skinless chicken breasts cut into 1-inch cubes

- • 2cups of water

- • ¼ of the red bell pepper cut into 1-inch thick strips

Directions:

1. In a heavy-bottomed pot, heat oil on the medium-high fire.

2. Sauté garlic and ginger until garlic is starting to brown, around 1 to 2 minutes.

3. Add curry, turmeric, cinnamon, clove, bay leaf, and fenugreek. Sauté until fragrant, around 3 to 5 minutes.

4. Add tomatoes and onions. Sauté for 5 to ten minutes or until tomatoes are wilted, and onions are soft and translucent. If needed, add ¼ cup of water.

5. Add chicken breasts and sauté for 5 minutes—season with pepper and salt.

6. Add remaining water; bring to a boil, then slow fire to medium. While covered, continue cooking chicken for at least 15 minutes.

7. Add bell pepper and coconut milk. Cook until heated through.

8. Turn off fire and serve best with brown rice.

Nutrition:

Calories 225, Total Fat 8g, Saturated Fat 1.6g, Total Carbs 12g, Net Carbs 10g, Protein 28g, Sugar: 4g, Fiber 2g, Sodium 1290mg, Potassium 782mg

Turkey And Quinoa Stuffed Peppers

Preparation Time: 15 minutes

Cooking time: 35 minutes

Servings: 6

Ingredients:

- Three large red bell peppers
- 2tsp chopped fresh rosemary
- 2tbsp chopped fresh parsley
- 3tbsp chopped pecans, toasted
- 2 tbsp. extra virgin olive oil
- ½ cup chicken stock
- ½ lb. fully cooked smoked turkey sausage, diced
- ½ tsp. salt
- 2cups of water
- 1cup uncooked quinoa

Directions:

1. On high fire, place a large saucepan and add salt, water, and quinoa. Bring to a boil.

2. Once boiling, reduce fire to a simmer, cover, and cook until all water is absorbed, around 15 minutes.

3. Uncover quinoa, turn off the fire, and let it stand for another 5 minutes.

4. Add rosemary, parsley, pecans, olive oil, chicken stock, and turkey sausage into quinoa pan. Mix well.

5. Slice peppers lengthwise in half and discards membranes and seeds. In another boiling pot of water, add peppers, boil for 5 minutes, drain and discard water.

6. Grease a 13 x 9 baking dish and preheat oven to 350oF.

7. Place boiled bell pepper onto a prepared baking dish, evenly fill with the quinoa mixture, and pop into the oven.

8. Bake for 15 minutes.

Nutrition:

Calories 253, Total Fat 13g, Saturated Fat 2g, Total Carbs 21g, Net Carbs 19.7g, Protein 14g, Sugar: 1.3g, Fiber 3g, Sodium 545mg, Potassium 372mg

Curried Chicken, Chickpeas And Raita Salad

Preparation Time: 10 minutes

Cooking time: 30 minutes

Servings: 5

Ingredients:

- 1cup red grapes halved
- 3-4cups rotisserie chicken, meat coarsely shredded
- 2tbsp cilantro
- 1cup plain yogurt
- Two medium tomatoes, chopped
- 1tsp ground cumin
- 1tbsp curry powder
- 2tbsp vegetable oil
- 1tbsp minced peeled ginger
- 1tbsp minced garlic

- One medium onion, chopped

Chickpeas Ingredients:

- ¼ tsp. cayenne

- ½ tsp. turmeric

- 1tsp ground cumin

- one 19-oz can chickpeas, rinsed, drained, and patted dry

- 1tbsp vegetable oil

Topping and Raita Ingredients:

½ cup sliced and toasted almonds

2tbsp chopped mint

2cups cucumber, peeled, cored, and chopped

1cup plain yogurt

Directions:

1. To make the chicken salad, place a medium nonstick saucepan and heat oil on a medium-low fire.

2. Sauté ginger, garlic, and onion for 5 minutes or until softened while stirring occasionally.

3. Add 1 ½ tsp.: salt, cumin, and curry. Sauté
   for two minutes.

4. Increase fire to medium-high and add
   tomatoes. Stirring frequently, cook for 5
   minutes.

5. Pour sauce into a bowl, mix in chicken,
   cilantro, and yogurt. Stir to combine and
   let it stand to cool to room temperature.

6. To make the chickpeas, on a nonstick fry
   pan, heat oil for 3 minutes.

7. Add chickpeas and cook for a minute while
   stirring frequently.

8. Add ¼ tsp.: salt, cayenne, turmeric, and
   cumin. Stir to mix well and cook for two
   minutes or until sauce is dried.

9. Transfer to a bowl and let it cool to room
   temperature.

10. To make the raita, mix ½ tsp.: salt,
    mint, cucumber, and yogurt. Stir
    thoroughly to combine and dissolve the
    salt.

11. In four 16-oz lidded jars or bowls, to assemble, layer the following: curried chicken, raita, chickpeas, and garnish with almonds.

12. You can make this recipe one day ahead and refrigerate for 6 hours before serving.

Nutrition:

Calories 403, Total Fat 16g, Saturated Fat 3g, Total Carbs 42g, Net Carbs 33g, Protein 26g, Sugar: 17g, Fiber 9g, Sodium 312mg, Potassium 747mg

Balsamic Vinaigrette On Roasted Chicken

Preparation Time: 10 minutes

Cooking time: 60 minutes

Servings: 8

Ingredients:

- 1tbsp chopped fresh parsley
- 1tsp lemon zest
- ½ cup low-salt chicken broth
- One 4-lb whole chicken, cut into pieces
- Freshly ground black pepper
- Salt
- 2tbsp olive oil
- Two garlic cloves, chopped
- 2tbsp fresh lemon juice
- 2tbsp Dijon mustard
- ¼ cup balsamic vinegar

Directions:

1. In a small bowl, whisk to blend pepper, salt, olive oil, garlic, lemon juice, mustard, and vinegar.

2. In a re-sealable bag, combine the above mixture and chicken pieces. Refrigerate and marinate for at least 2 hours to a whole day. Ensure to turn the bag upside down occasionally.

3. Grease a baking dish and preheat the oven to 400oF.

4. Arrange marinated chicken pieces onto a baking dish and pop into the oven.

5. Roast chicken for an hour. If chicken is browned and not yet fully cooked, cover with foil and continue cooking.

6. Remove from oven, and transfer chicken to a serving plate.

7. Garnish with parsley and drizzle with lemon juice before serving.

Nutrition:

Calories 296, Total Fat 10g, Saturated Fat 2g, Total Carbs 2g, Net Carbs 1.8g, Protein 47g, Sugar: 1.4g, Fiber 0.2g, Sodium 278mg, Potassium 580mg

Chicken Pasta Parmesan

Preparation Time: 10 minutes

Cooking time: 20 minutes

Servings: 1

Ingredients:

- ½ cup cooked whole-wheat spaghetti
- 1oz reduced-fat mozzarella cheese, grated
- ¼ cup prepared marinara sauce
- 2tbsp seasoned dry breadcrumbs
- 4oz skinless chicken breast
- 1tbsp olive oil

Directions:

1. On medium-high fire, place an ovenproof skillet and heat oil.

2. Pan Fry chicken for 3 to 5 minutes per side or until cooked through.

3. Pour marinara sauce, stir and continue cooking for 3 minutes.

4. Turn off the fire; add mozzarella and breadcrumbs on top.

5. Pop into a preheated broiler on high and broil for 10 minutes or until breadcrumbs are browned, and mozzarella is melted.

6. Remove from broiler, serve, and enjoy.

Nutrition:

Calories 492, Total Fat 19g, Saturated Fat 3g, Total Carbs 32g, Net Carbs 21g, Protein 49g, Sugar: 11g, Fiber 6g, Sodium 488mg, Potassium 605mg

Chicken And White Bean

Preparation Time: 10 minutes

Cooking time: 70 minutes

Servings: 6

Ingredients:

- 2tbsp fresh cilantro, chopped
- 2cups grated low-fat Monterey Jack cheese
- 3cups of water
- 1/8 tsp. cayenne pepper
- 2tsp pure Chile powder
- 2tsp ground cumin
- One 4-oz can be chopped green chilies
- 1cup corn kernels
- Two 15-oz cans of white beans drained and rinsed
- Two garlic cloves
- One medium onion, diced

- • 2tbsp extra virgin olive oil

- • 1lb. chicken breasts, boneless and skinless

Directions:

1. Slice chicken breasts into ½-inch cubes, and with pepper and salt, season it.

2. On high fire, place a large nonstick fry pan and heat oil.

3. Sauté chicken pieces for three to four minutes or until lightly browned.

4. Reduce fire to medium and add garlic and onion.

5. Cook for 5 to 6 minutes or until onions is translucent.

6. Add water, spices, chilies, corn, and beans. Bring to a boil.

7. Once boiling, slow fire to a simmer and continue simmering for an hour, uncovered.

8. To serve, garnish with a sprinkling of cilantro and a tablespoon of cheese.

Nutrition:

Calories 550, Total Fat 18g, Saturated Fat 3g, Total Carbs 51g, Net Carbs 37g, Protein 48g, Sugar: 2g, Fiber 14g, Sodium 817mg, Potassium 1282mg

Chicken Pad Thai

Preparation Time: 10 minutes

Cooking time: 10 minutes

Servings: 6

Ingredients:

- Two medium-sized carrots, julienned
- One 12oz package broccoli slaw
- Five green onions, chopped
- 5tbsp fresh cilantro, chopped
- ½ tbsp. coconut vinegar
- 4tbsp fresh lime juice
- 1tbsp coconut amino
- 3tbsp fish sauce
- Five cloves garlic, crushed
- 2tbsp extra virgin coconut oil
- 1½ lb. organic chicken meat, cut into chunks

Directions:

1. Heat the skillet over medium-high heat and add the coconut oil.

2. Sauté the garlic and onion for one minute.

3. Add the chicken and cook for five minutes.

4. Add the coconut amino, fish sauce, vinegar, and lime juice. Increase the heat to high and simmer until the chicken is thoroughly cooked.

5. Add the broccoli slaw and carrots. Stir constantly until the vegetables become soft.

6. Garnish with cilantro and green onions.

Nutrition:

Calories 287, Total Fat 10g, Saturated Fat 2.2g, Total Carbs 10g, Net Carbs 8g, Protein 38g, Sugar: 4g, Fiber 2g, Sodium 836mg, Potassium 683mg